PANCREATITIS DIET COOKBOOK FOR DOGS

Quick & Easy Homemade Recipes to Heal and Manage Pancreatitis

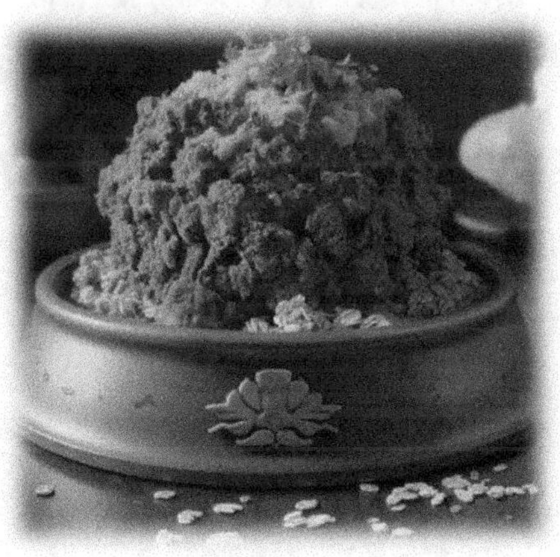

DR. MUTEER CALVIN

TABLE OF CONTENTS

INTRODUCTION 4

WHAT IS PANCREATITIS? 6

What Is Pancreatitis in Dogs? 6

Causes of Pancreatitis in Dogs 6

Symptoms of Pancreatitis in Dogs................... 7

TREATMENT REQUIRED 9

Treatment for Pancreatitis in Dogs................... 9

Role of Diet in Managing Pancreatitis in Dogs. ..12

Dietary Management of Pancreatitis in Dogs12

PANCREATITIS DIETS FOR DOGS................. 15

Conclusion 85

INTRODUCTION

Welcome to the "Pancreatitis Diet Cookbook for Dogs

If you're reading this, it's likely that you're a dog owner who has had to grapple with the reality of your beloved pet being diagnosed with pancreatitis. It's a tough pill to swallow, but remember, you're not alone. This book is a testament to the love and dedication that we, as pet parents, have for our furry friends.

This cookbook is more than just a collection of recipes. It's a comprehensive guide designed to help you navigate the often confusing world of canine pancreatitis. It's a resource that will empower you to take control of your dog's health through the most fundamental aspect of their lives - their diet.

In the following pages, you'll find a wealth of information on what pancreatitis is, how it affects your dog, and most importantly, how you can manage it through proper nutrition. You'll discover a variety of recipes that are not only safe for dogs with pancreatitis but are also delicious and easy to prepare. These recipes have been carefully crafted to ensure they meet the nutritional needs of dogs suffering from this condition, helping them recover and thrive.

But this book isn't just about the food. It's about giving you the knowledge and confidence to care for your dog in the best way possible. It's about providing you with peace of mind knowing that you're doing everything you can to help your dog live a happy, healthy life.

So, whether you're new to the world of canine pancreatitis or you've been dealing with it for a while, this book is for you. Let's embark on this journey together, for the love of our dogs.

Welcome to the "Pancreatitis Diet Cookbook for Dogs".

WHAT IS PANCREATITIS?

What Is Pancreatitis in Dogs?

Inflammation of the pancreas is a symptom of pancreatitis. Adjacent to your dog's stomach, the pancreas is an organ that makes insulin to control blood sugar and digestive enzymes to help in digestion.

These enzymes don't start working in a healthy dog until they get to the small intestine. On the other hand, early activation of the enzymes results in inflammation and damage to the surrounding tissue and pancreas in dogs suffering from pancreatitis. In extreme situations, the pancreas itself may start to be digested by the enzymes, producing excruciating pain.

Causes of Pancreatitis in Dogs

A common cause of pancreatitis is dietary errors, such as consuming something improperly. This might be as a result of them finding a fatty treat at the park, getting into the trash, or eating a lot of table leftovers. It can, nevertheless, also happen seemingly out of the blue.

Symptoms of Pancreatitis in Dogs

Depending on whether a dog's pancreatitis is acute (with a fast onset) or chronic (develops over time), the symptoms can change.

These are a few typical symptoms:

Excessive Fatigue: Dogs suffering from pancreatitis frequently exhibit excessive fatigue and reluctance to move.

Abdominal Pain: Pain or distention of the abdomen is a common symptom. Your dog may look bloated or uncomfortable.

Persistent Vomiting: This can happen multiple times in a few hours or on occasion over several days.

Diarrhea: Diarrhea can occur in some dogs with pancreatitis.

Loss of Appetite or Refusal to Eat: Dogs with pancreatitis frequently lose their appetite.

Dehydration: This can happen if your dog has been vomiting or has diarrhea.

Fever: Some dogs with pancreatitis may experience fever.

In the event that your dog displays any number of these symptoms, it's critical to seek veterinary attention as soon as possible, particularly if the symptoms are severe or last longer than a day.

If pancreatitis is not treated quickly, it might worsen and cause other health issues.

Though you may find this material useful in understanding canine pancreatitis, you should always seek the opinion of a veterinarian for your pet's medical needs and available treatments.

TREATMENT REQUIRED

Treatment for Pancreatitis in Dogs

The cornerstone of managing acute pancreatitis in dogs is supportive care, which encompasses nutritional guidance and hydration therapy.

Here are a few crucial elements of the care:

1. Pain Management:

Dogs suffering from pancreatitis frequently endure excruciating pain. Usually, anti-inflammatory medications and painkillers are used to treat this pain.

In more severe situations, a customized, multimodal strategy to analgesia may be employed, involving the use of opioids, local anesthetic drugs, and/or NMDA (N-methyl-D-aspartate) antagonists like ketamine.

2. Hydration:

Two frequent symptoms of pancreatitis are vomiting and diarrhea, both of which can lead to dehydration. Intravenous fluids are frequently administered to address electrolyte imbalances and replenish dehydration.

3. Nutritional Management:

To give the pancreas a break, food and liquids may be denied for a whole day at first. Following this time, a prescription dog food that is low in fat, highly digestible, and bland is gradually added.

4. Medication:

You may also be given medication to address diarrhea and vomiting. Antibiotics may be used in certain situations.

5. Monitoring:

Throughout the course of treatment, regular monitoring is essential. This enables the veterinarian to monitor for any issues and modify the treatment routine as needed.

6. Hospitalization:

Intensive hospitalization may be necessary for more severe cases of pancreatitis.

Aggressive supportive care, such as dietary management, analgesia, antiemetics, gastrointestinal acid suppression, and correction of abnormalities related to fluid, electrolyte, and acid-base balance, is included in this.

Recall that pancreatitis is a dangerous illness that may be fatal. It's critical to get your dog checked out by a veterinarian as soon as you suspect pancreatitis.

Role of Diet in Managing Pancreatitis in Dogs.

Dietary Management of Pancreatitis in Dogs

When it comes to treating pancreatitis in dogs, nutrition is thought to be crucial. The following are some crucial nutritional management elements:

1. Low-Fat Diet:

In the past, fat was thought to be the main nutrient that was important in pancreatitis. In dogs, low-fat gastrointestinal diets are often advised during the first stages of pancreatitis management. Long-term use of a low-fat diet may be recommended for dogs that experience repeated pancreatitis episodes.

2. Protein and Carbohydrates:

In these situation, other nutrients and dietary components, such as protein and carbohydrates, are also crucial. As for managing pancreatitis in dogs, it's possible that protein particle size matters more than dietary fat.

3. Hydrolyzed Diets:

First-line diets for dogs with pancreatitis are frequently hydrolyzed diets, because they consist of smaller-component proteins.

4. Enteral Nutrition:

Enteral nutrition is typically a part of nutritional support, which is a therapeutic role in the care of dogs with acute pancreatitis. Feeding a dog with a tube that enters the stomach or small intestine directly is known as enteral nutrition. The benefits of early enteral nutrition are now strongly advocated above parenteral nutrition for the majority of cases in dogs with pancreatitis, notwithstanding the paucity of studies in this area.

5. Transitioning Back to Regular Diet:

If there is no substantial coexisting condition, many dogs with pancreatitis can return to their pre-diagnosis diet or another commercial maintenance diet.

PANCREATITIS DIETS FOR DOGS

1. Turkey and Sweet Potato Stew:

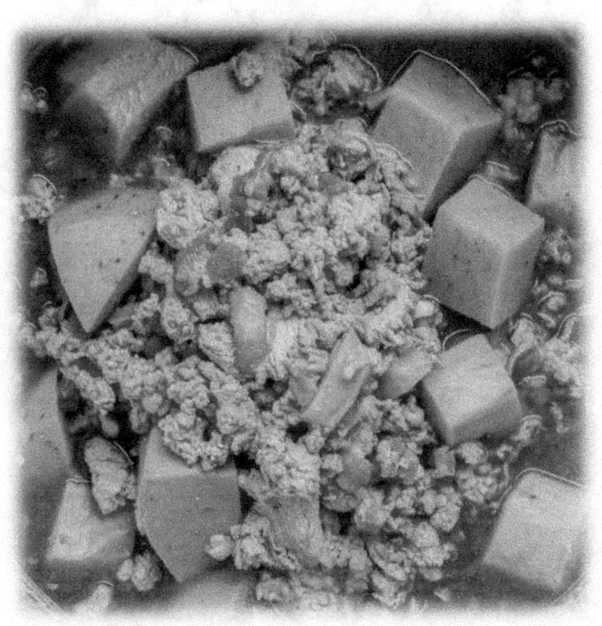

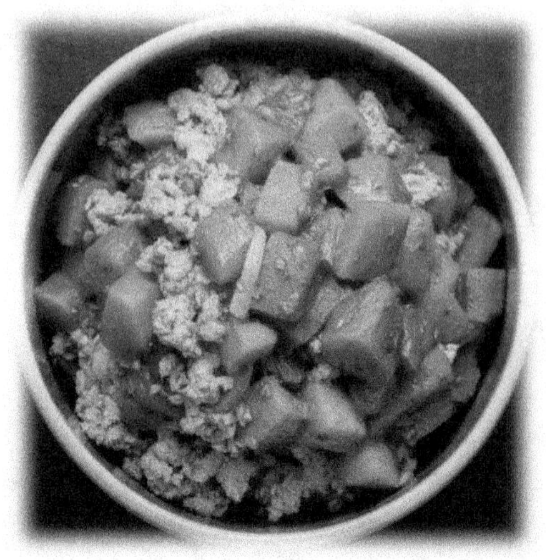

Ingredients:

1 pound, Lean Ground Turkey

2 sweet potatoes, chopped and peeled

4 cups low sodium chicken broth

Instructions:

1. Over medium heat, brown the ground turkey in a large pot.

2. Include the chicken broth and chopped sweet potatoes. Sweet potatoes should be simmered for 20-25 minutes until soft.

3. Serve once cooled to room temperature.

2. Chicken and Rice Casserole:

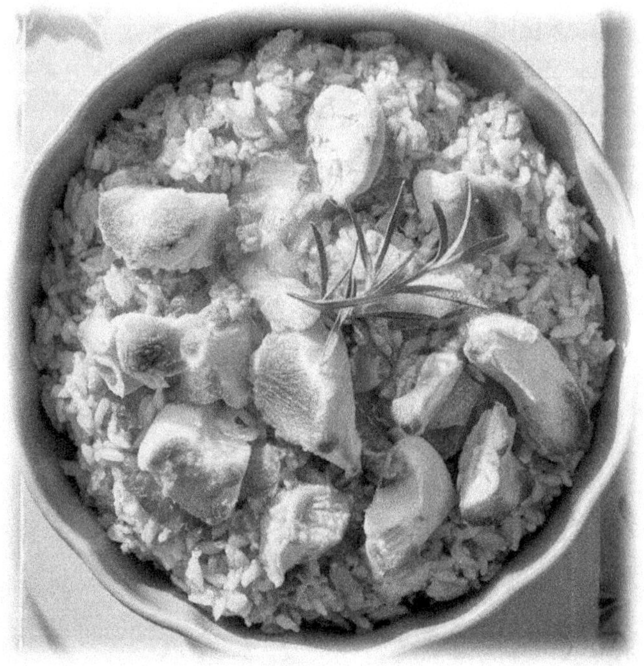

Ingredients:

1 pound of diced, skinless, boneless chicken breast

2 cups of cooked brown rice

1 cup of Low sodium chicken broth

Instructions:

1. Set oven temperature to 175°C/350°F.

2. Put cooked brown rice, chicken broth, and diced chicken into a baking dish.

3. Bake the chicken for 25-30 minutes, or until it's cooked through.

4. Let it cool before serving.

3. Fish and Quinoa Salad:

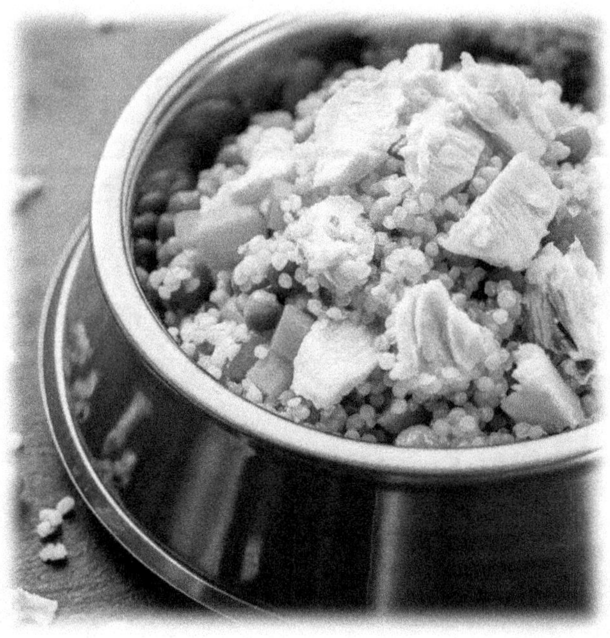

Ingredients:

1 pound of white fish fillets, such as cod or tilapia

1 cup of cooked quinoa

1 cup of mixed vegetables, such as peas and carrots

Instructions:

1. Bake or steam the fish until it's cooked.

2. Flake the fish and mix it with mixed vegetables and cooked quinoa.

3. Serve at room temperature.

4. Beef and Pumpkin Stew:

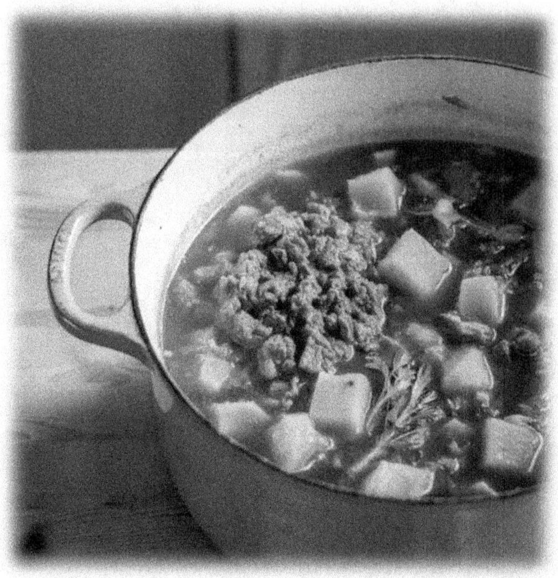

Ingredients:

1 pound of lean ground beef

1 cup of canned pumpkin (not pumpkin pie filling)

2 cups low-sodium beef broth

Instructions:

1. Brown the ground beef in a big pot over medium heat.

2. Add the beef broth and canned pumpkin. Give it a 20–25 minute simmer.

3. Let it cool before serving.

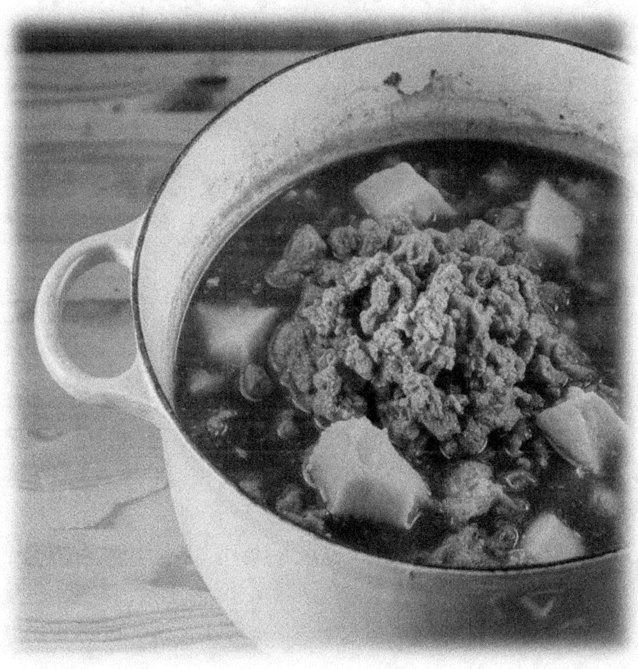

5. Turkey and Barley Soup:

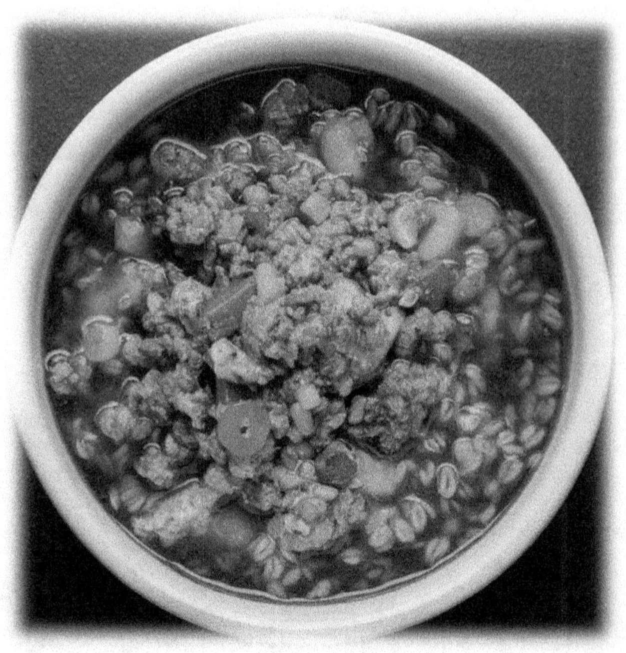

Ingredients:

1 pound of ground turkey

1 cup of cooked barley

4 cups of low sodium chicken broth

Instructions:

1. Over medium heat, brown the ground turkey in a large pot.

2. Add the chicken broth and cooked barley. Give it a 20–25 minute simmer.

3. Serve after chilled.

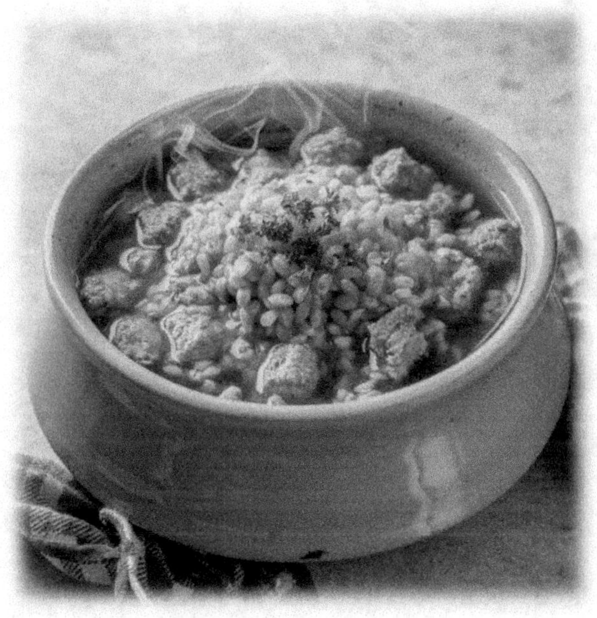

6. Chicken and Oatmeal Porridge:

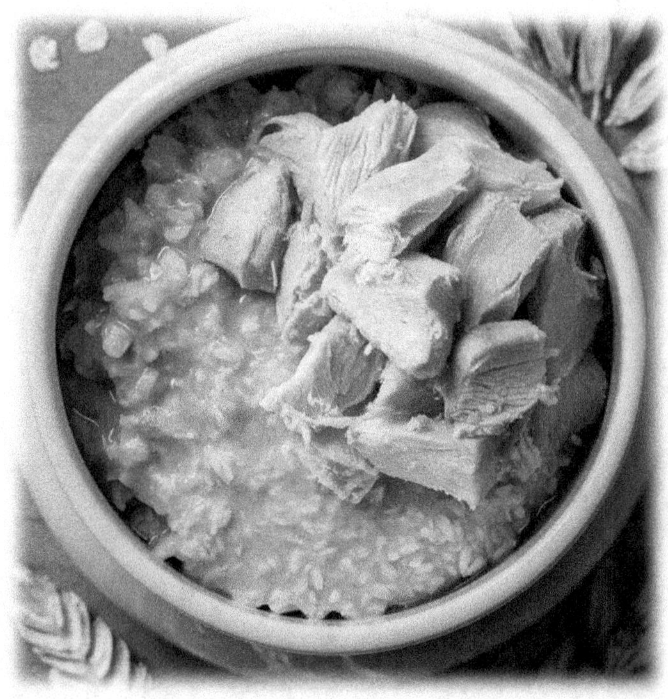

Ingredients:

1 pound of chopped, skinless, boneless chicken thighs

1 cup of cooked, plain, unsweetened oatmeal

2 cups of water

Instructions:

1. Cook chopped chicken thighs in water in a saucepan until done.

2. Add the cooked oats and simmer for a further 5 minutes.

3. Let it cool before serving.

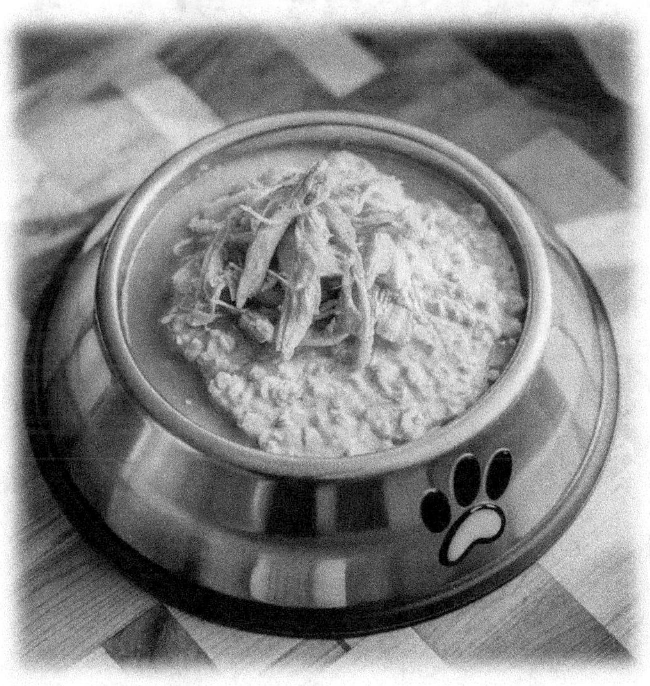

7. Fish and Potato Skillet:

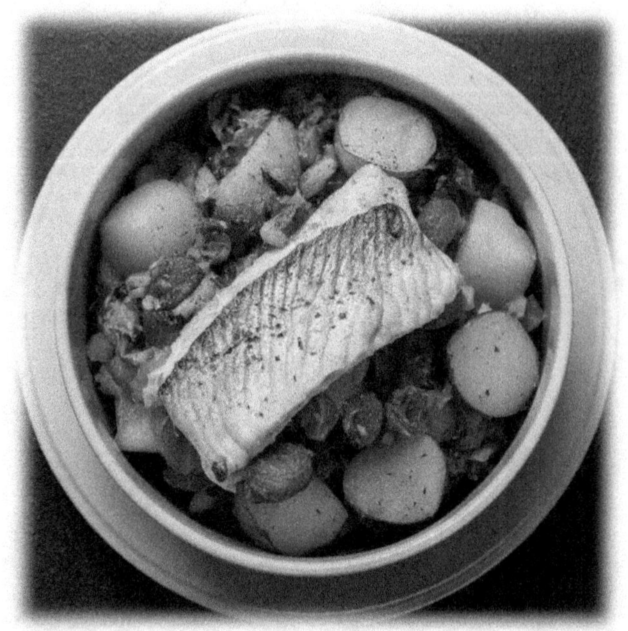

Ingredients:

1 pound of white fish fillets

2 potatoes, chopped and peeled

2 tablespoons of olive oil

Instructions:

1. Heat the olive oil in a skillet over medium heat.

2. Cook the diced potatoes until they become soft.

3. Add the fish fillets and cook them until they are flaky and opaque.

4. Serve after chilled.

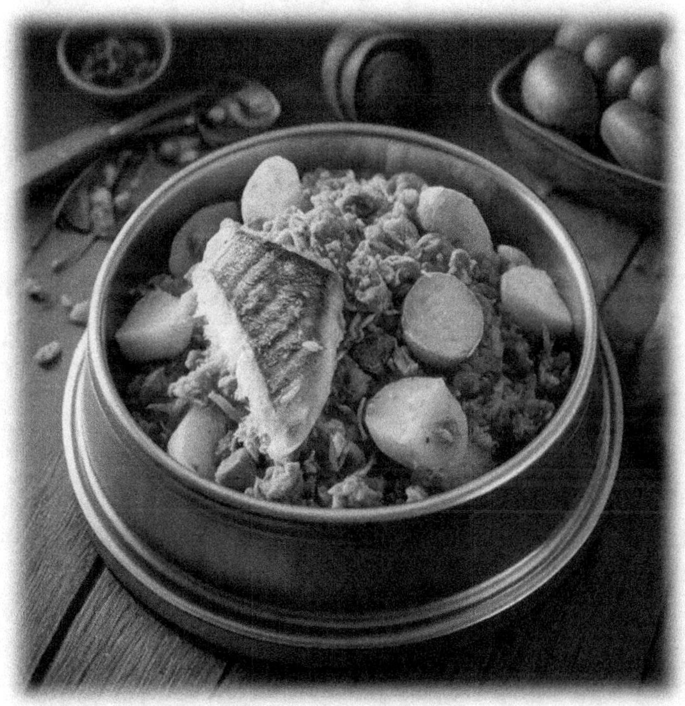

8. Venison and Rice Stir-Fry:

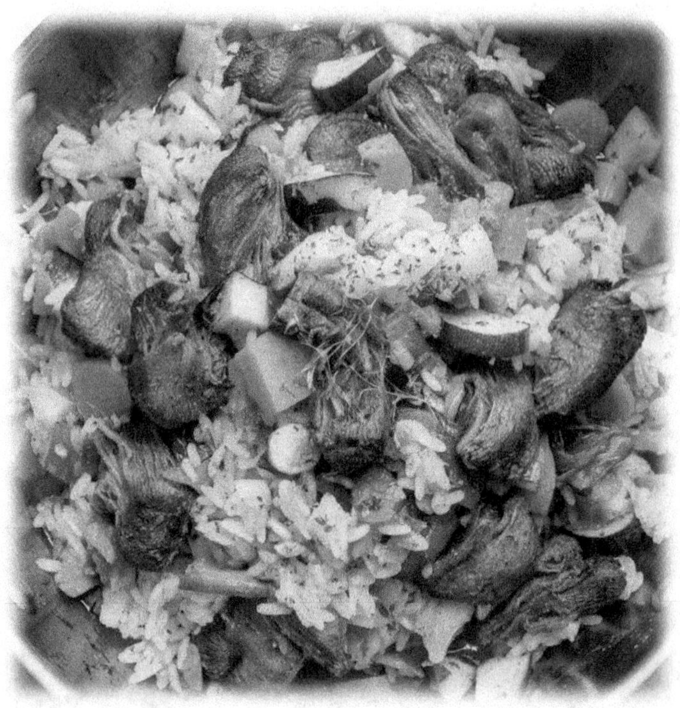

Ingredients:

1 pound of thinly sliced venison meat

2 cups of cooked white rice

1 cup of mixed vegetables, such as broccoli and bell peppers

Instructions:

1. Cook thinly sliced venison meat in a stir-fry until it's done.

2. Add mixed vegetables and cooked white rice. Sauté the vegetable until they are soft.

3. Let it cool before serving.

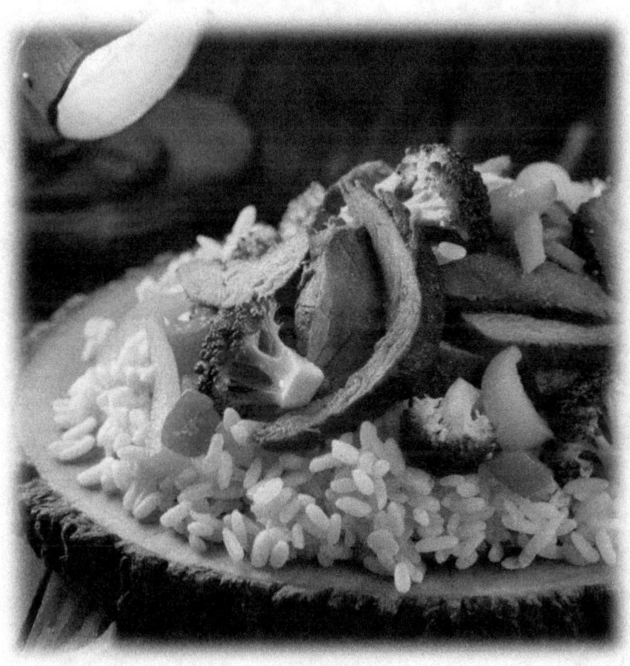

9. Lamb and Lentil Casserole:

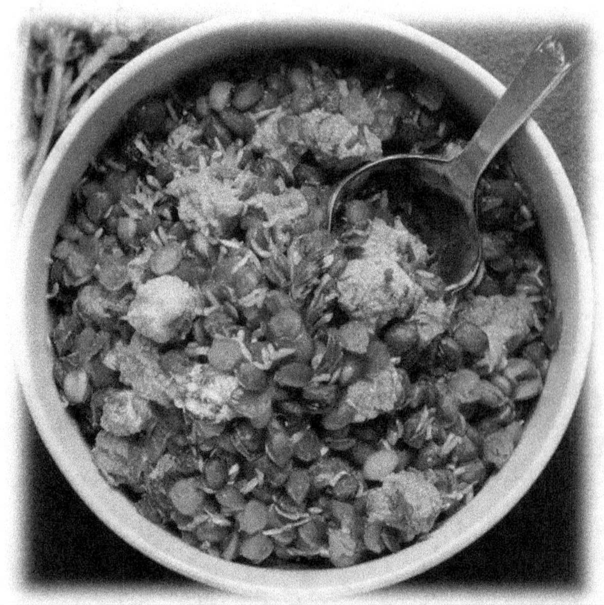

Ingredients:

1 pound of chopped lean lamb meat

1 cup of cooked lentils

2 cups low sodium lamb broth

Instructions:

1. Combine cooked lentils, diced lamb meat, and lamb broth in a baking dish.

2. Bake the lamb for 30-35 minutes at 350°F/175°C, or until it is cooked.

3. Serve after chilled.

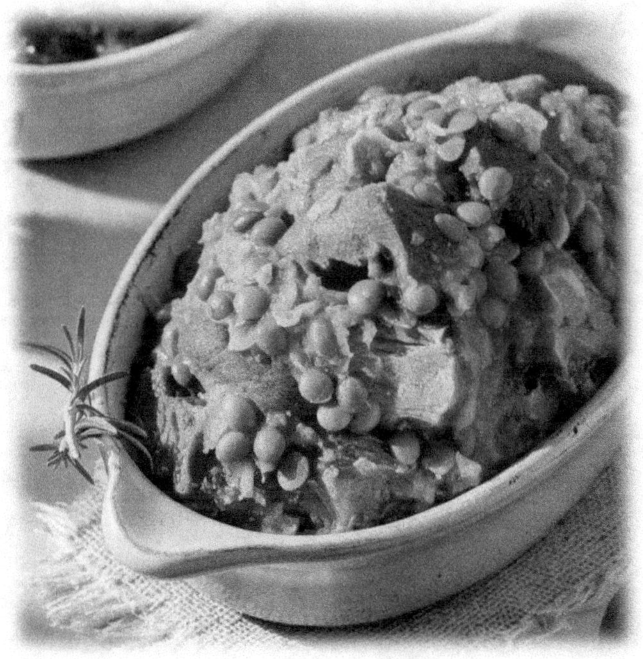

10. Chicken and Pumpkin Mash:

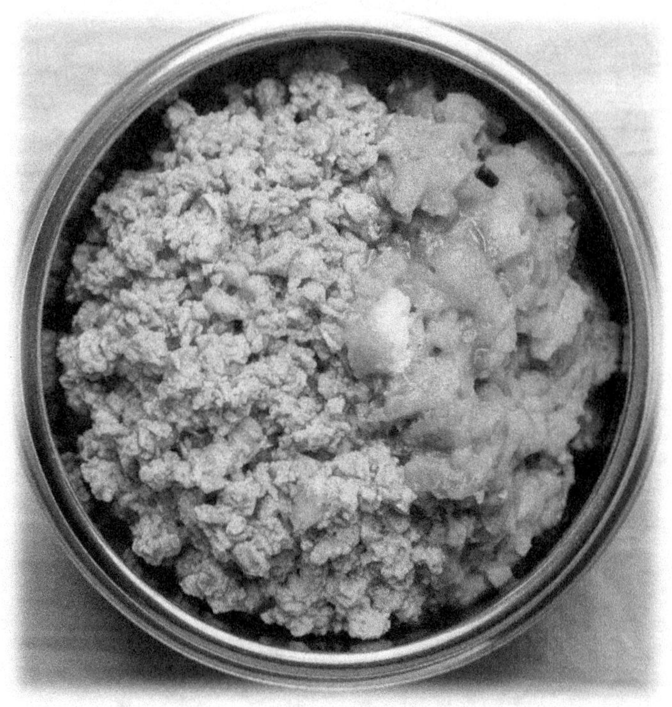

Ingredients:

1 pound of skinless, boneless chicken breasts

1 cup of canned pumpkin (not pumpkin pie filling)

1 tablespoon of coconut oil

Instructions:

1. Cook chicken breasts through by poaching them in water.

2. Shred the cooked chicken and combine it with coconut oil and canned pumpkin.

3. Mash to a smooth consistency and serve chilled.

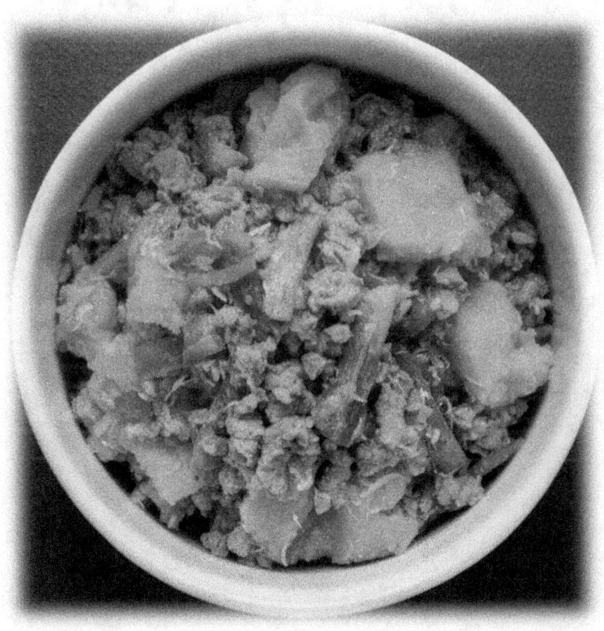

11. Turkey and Rice Congee:

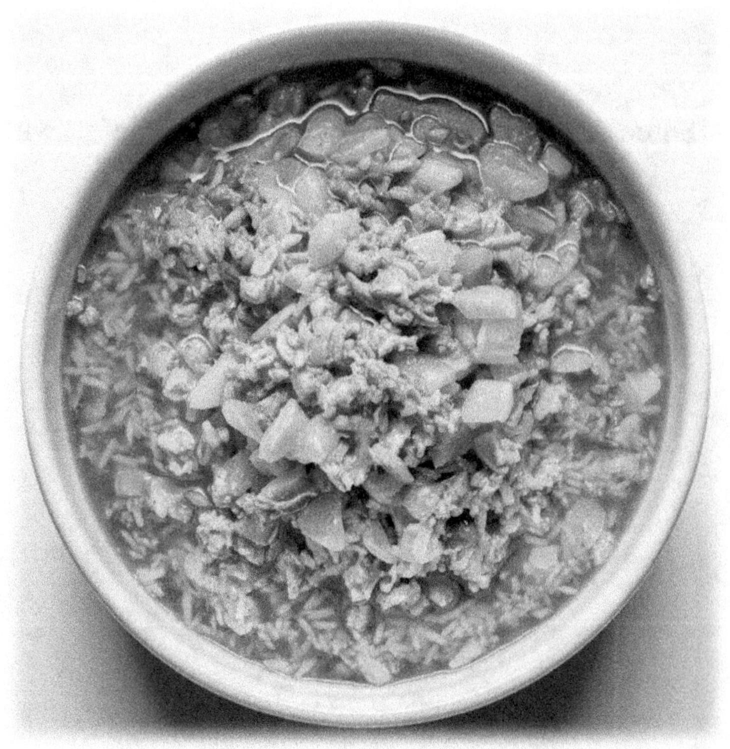

Ingredients:

1 cup of white rice

1 pound of ground turkey

4 cups low sodium chicken broth

Instructions:

1. In a pot, cook the ground turkey until browned.

2. Add the chicken broth and white rice. Simmer until the mixture thickens and the rice is done.

3. Let it cool before serving.

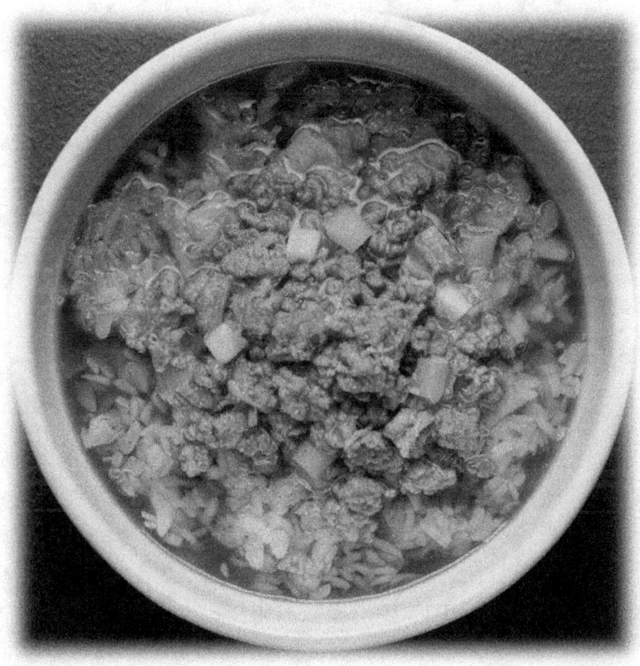

12. Chicken and Carrot Medley:

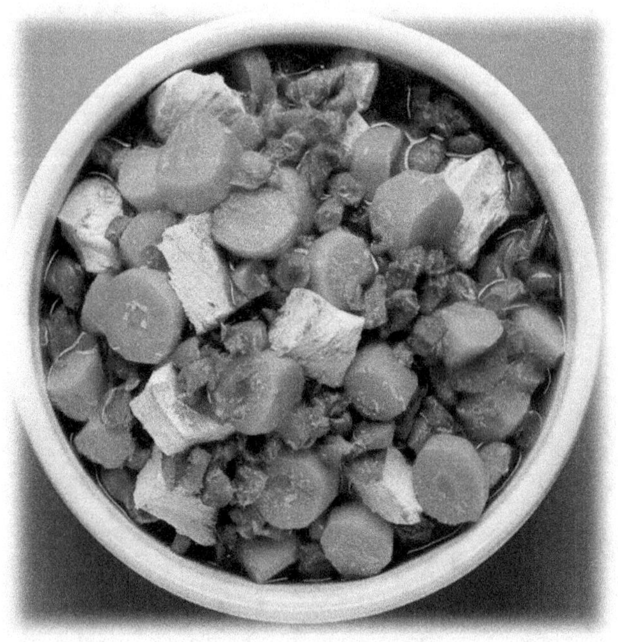

Ingredients:

1 pound of diced, skinless, boneless chicken thighs

2 cups of chopped carrots

1 cup of low sodium chicken broth

Instructions:

1. Cook chicken thighs thoroughly in a skillet.

2. Add the chicken broth and sliced carrots. Cook carrots until they become soft.

3. Serve after chilled.

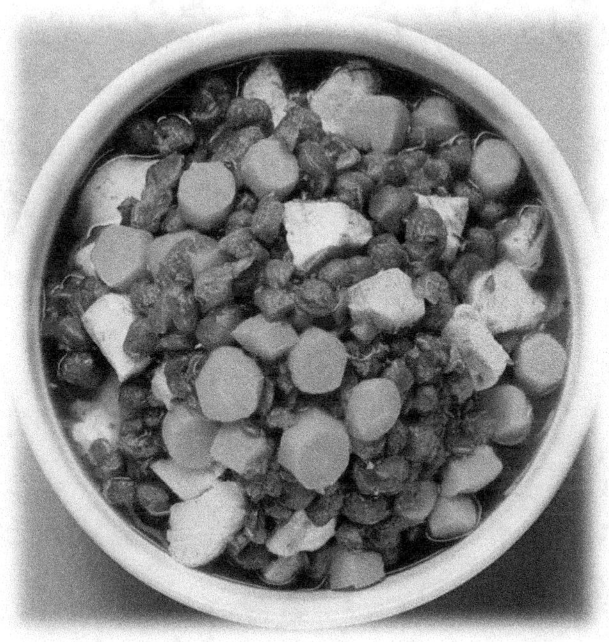

13. Fish and Spinach Bake:

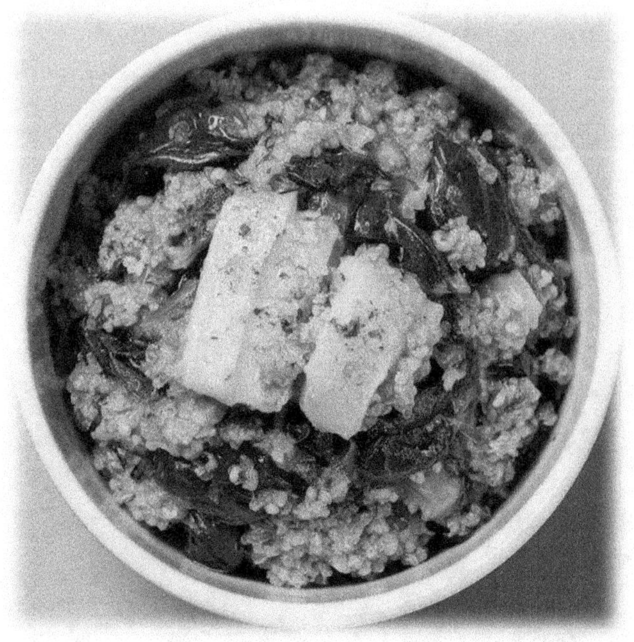

Ingredients:

1 pound of white fish fillets

2 cups of finely chopped spinach

1 cup of cooked quinoa

Instructions:

1. Fish fillets should be put on a baking dish.

2. Add cooked quinoa and chopped spinach on top.

3. Bake for 20-25 minutes or until the salmon flakes easily, at 375°F (190°C).

4. Let it cool before serving.

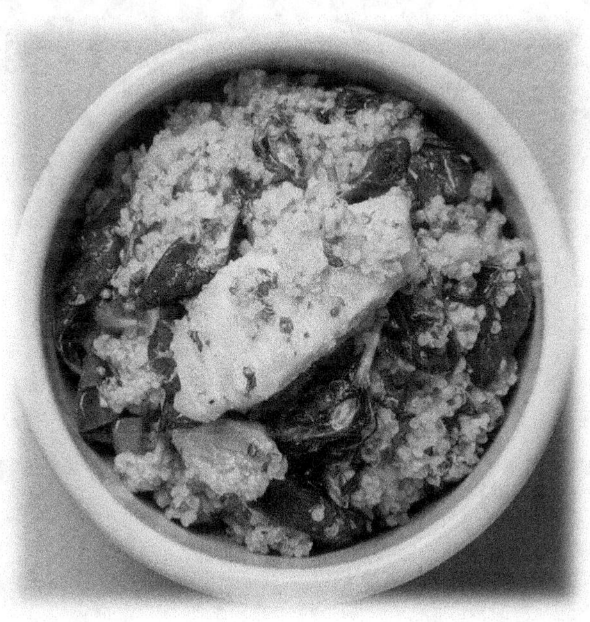

14. Turkey and Green Bean Stir-Fry:

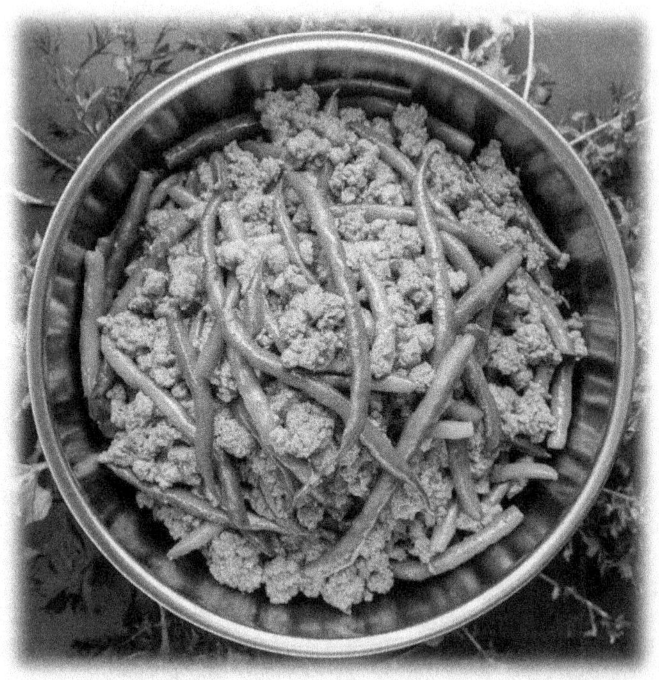

Ingredients:

1 pound of ground turkey

2 cups of finely chopped green beans

1 cup of cooked brown rice

Instructions:

1. In a skillet, cook the ground turkey until browned.

2. Add the cooked brown rice and diced green beans. Simmer the beans until they become soft.

3. Serve after chilled.

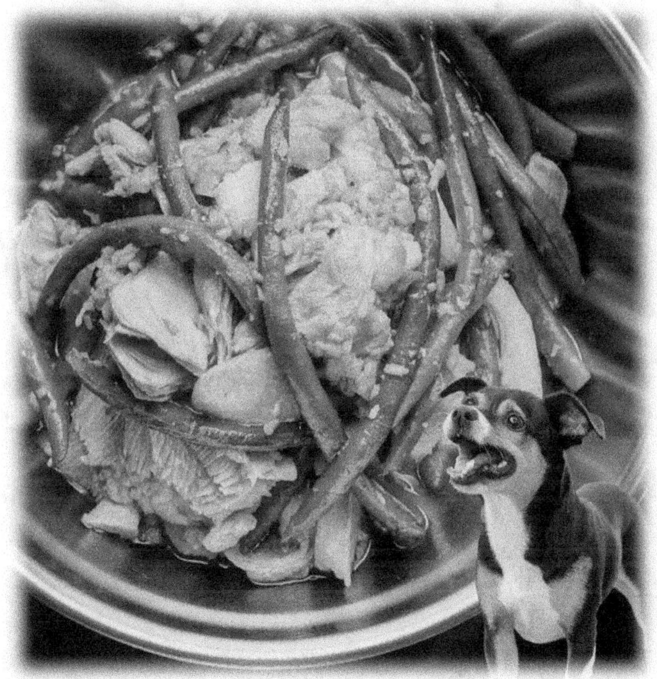

15. Chicken and Pea Casserole:

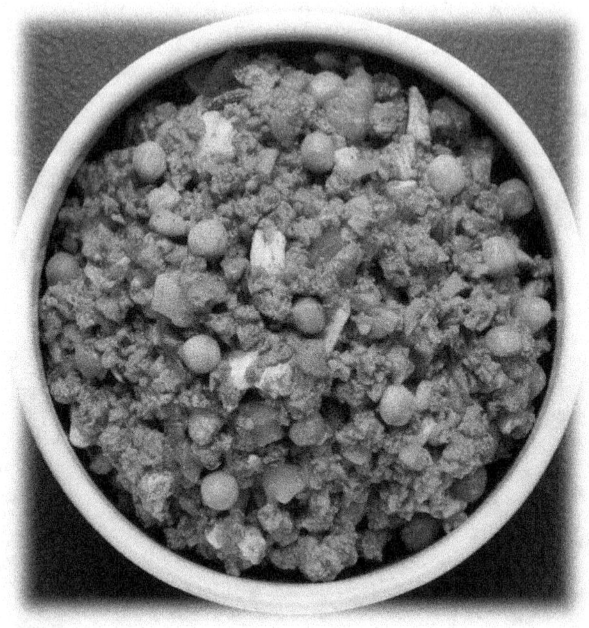

Ingredients:

1 pound of chopped, skinless, boneless chicken breasts

2 cups of fresh or frozen peas

1 cup of low sodium chicken broth

Instructions:

1. In a baking dish, mix together chopped chicken breasts, peas, and chicken broth.

2. Bake the chicken for 25-30 minutes, or until it is cooked through, at 350°F (175°C).

3. Let it cool before serving.

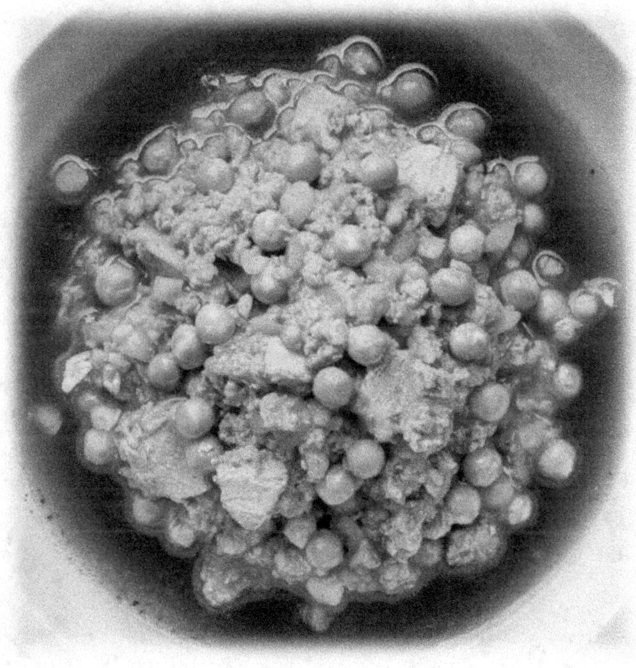

16. Beef and Carrot Stew:

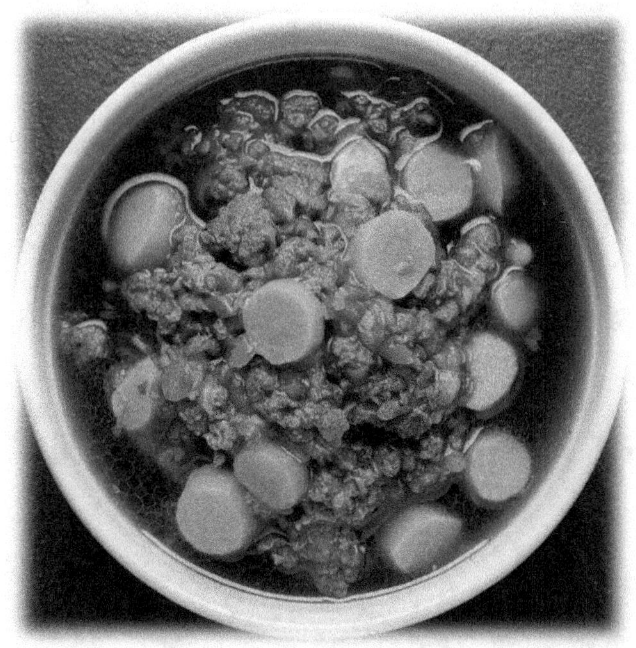

Ingredients:

1 pound of lean ground beef

2 cups of chopped carrots

2 cups low-sodium beef broth

Instructions:

1. In a pot over medium heat, brown the ground beef.

2. Add beef broth and chopped carrots. Carrots should simmer for 20-25 minutes to become soft.

3. Serve after chilled.

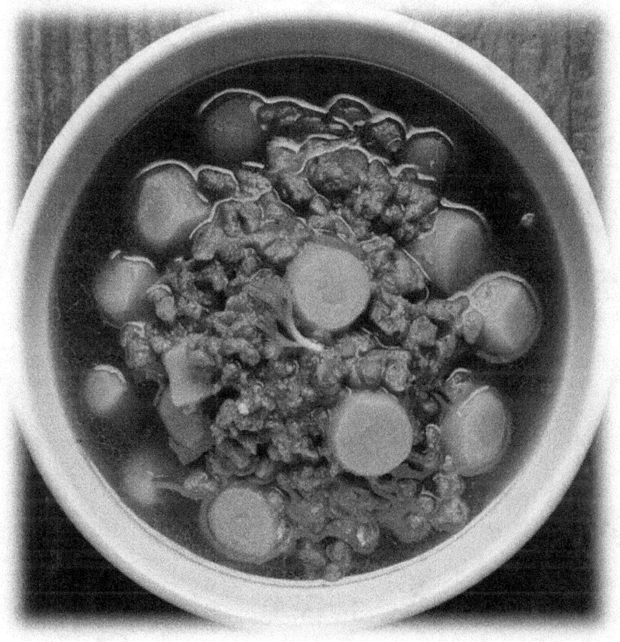

17. Salmon and Sweet Potato Mash:

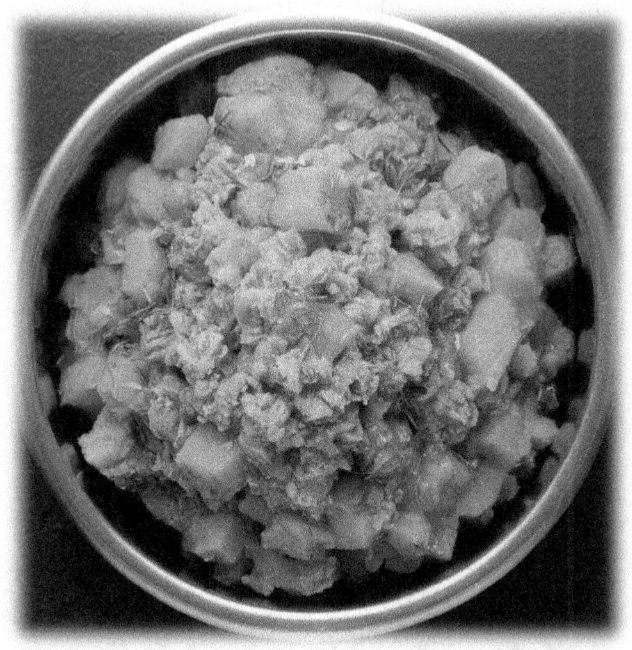

Ingredients:

1 pound of salmon fillets

2 cups of mashed sweet potatoes

1 tablespoon of olive oil

Instructions:

1. Cook the salmon fillets thoroughly in the oven.

2. Add olive oil, mashed sweet potatoes, and flaked cooked salmon to a mixture.

3. Serve at room temperature.

NB: You can ground the salmon fillet

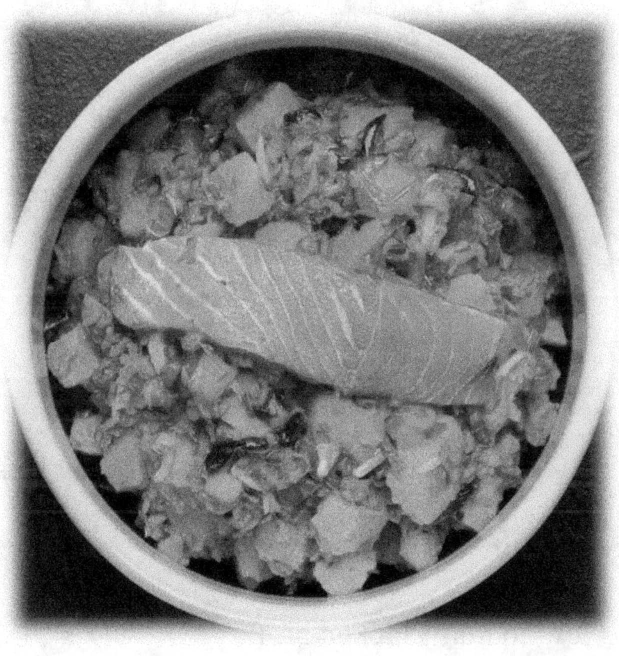

18. Chicken and Brown Rice Stew:

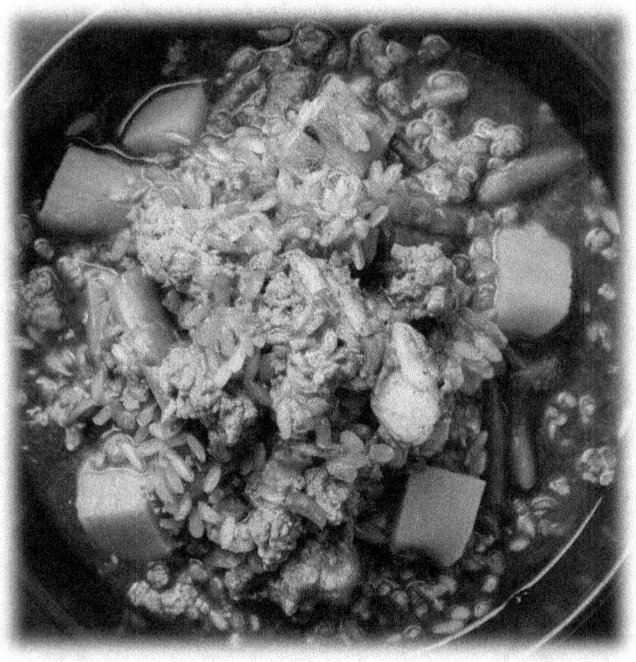

Ingredients:

1 pound of chopped boneless, skinless chicken thighs

2 cups cooked brown rice

4 cups low sodium chicken broth

Instructions:

1. Cook chopped chicken thighs in a pot until they are no longer pink.

2. Add the chicken broth and cooked brown rice. Give it a 20–25 minute simmer.

3. Let it cool before serving.

19. Turkey and Pumpkin Soup:

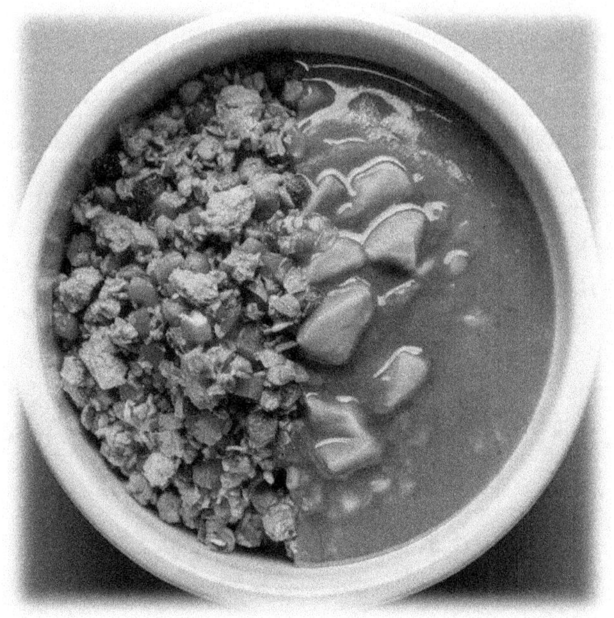

Ingredients:

1 pound of ground turkey

1 cup of canned pumpkin (not pumpkin pie filling)

4 cups low sodium turkey broth

Instructions:

1. In a large pot over medium heat, brown ground turkey.

2. Add the turkey broth and canned pumpkin. Give it a 20–25 minute simmer.

3. Serve after chilled.

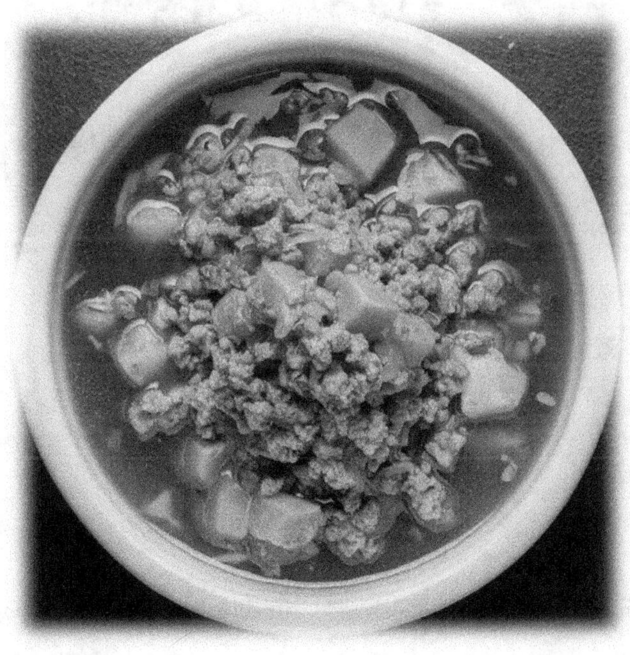

20. Lamb and Rice Pilaf:

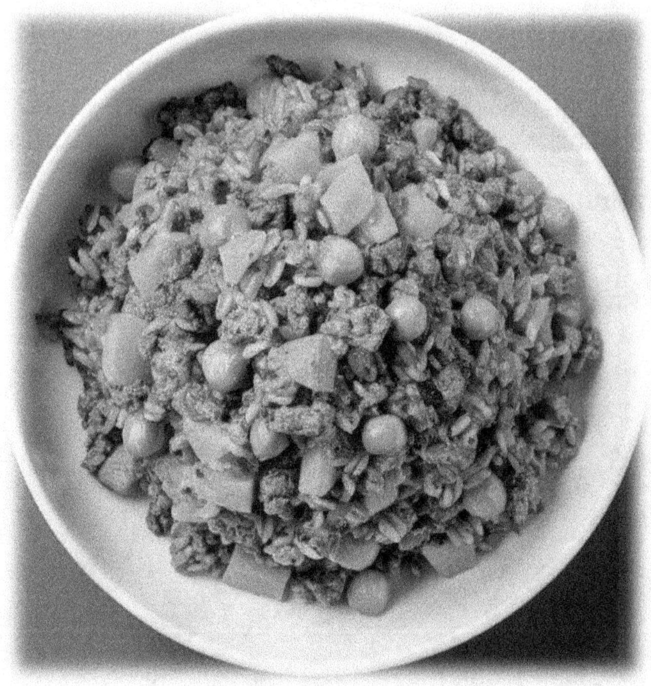

Ingredients:

1 pound of lean cubed lamb

2 cups of boiled white rice

1 cup of mixed vegetables, such as green beans and carrots

Instructions:

1. In a skillet, cook cubed lamb until browned.

2. Add mixed vegetables and cooked white rice. Sauté the veggies until they are soft.

3. Let it cool before serving.

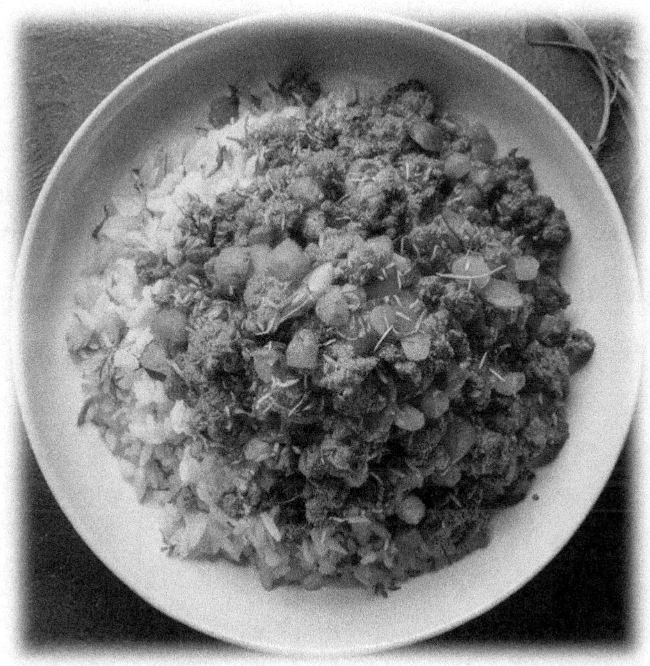

21. Chicken and Rice with Vegetables:

Ingredients:

1 cup of cooked chicken breast without bones or skin

½ cup of cooked white rice

½ cup chopped steamed green beans

¼ cup low-fat plain yogurt

Instructions:

1. Cook rice and chicken breast in separate pans.

2. Mix everything together and serve at room temperature.

22. Turkey and Sweet Potato:

Ingredients:

1 cup cooked sweet potato

1 cup cooked ground turkey

¼ cup chopped cooked carrots

1 tablespoon of pure canned pumpkin (pure not pie filling)

Instructions:

1. Cook the turkey and sweet potato separately.

2. Mix everything together and serve at room temperature.

23. White Fish and Oatmeal:

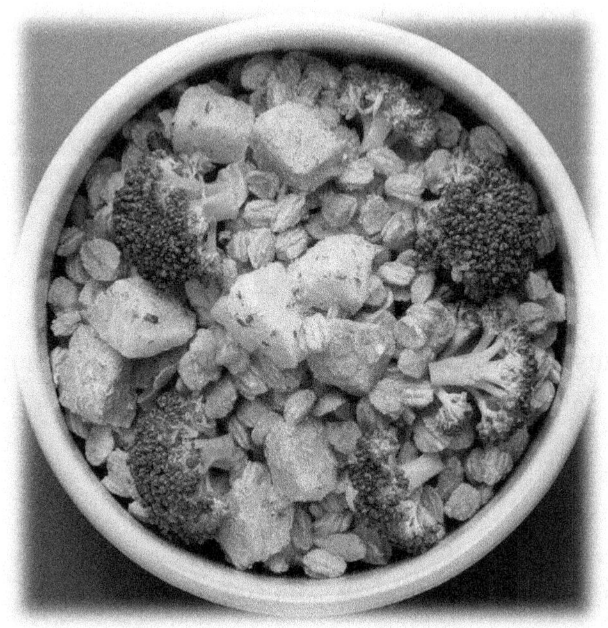

Ingredients:

1 cup cooked white fish (haddock, cod) without bones

½ cup of cooked oatmeal

¼ cup of cooked chopped broccoli florets

1 tablespoon of olive oil

Instructions:

1. Cook oatmeal and fish in separately.

2. Broccoli should be steamed until soft.

3. Mix everything together and serve at room temperature.

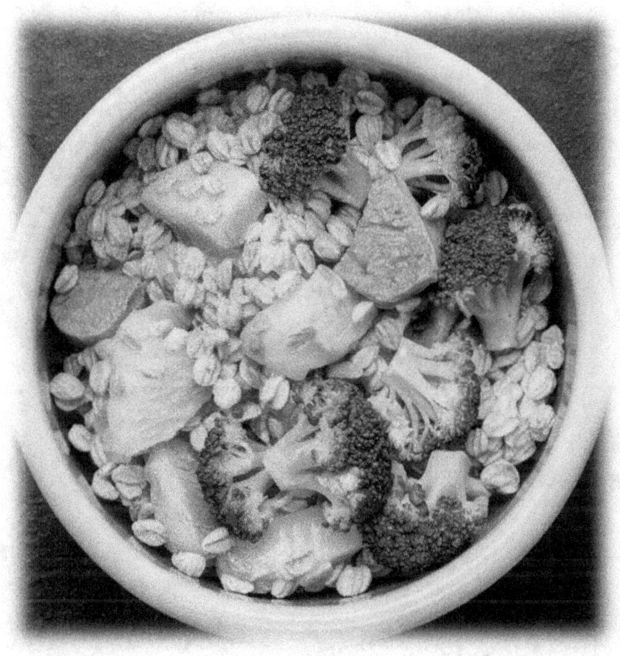

24. Cottage Cheese and Scrambled Eggs:

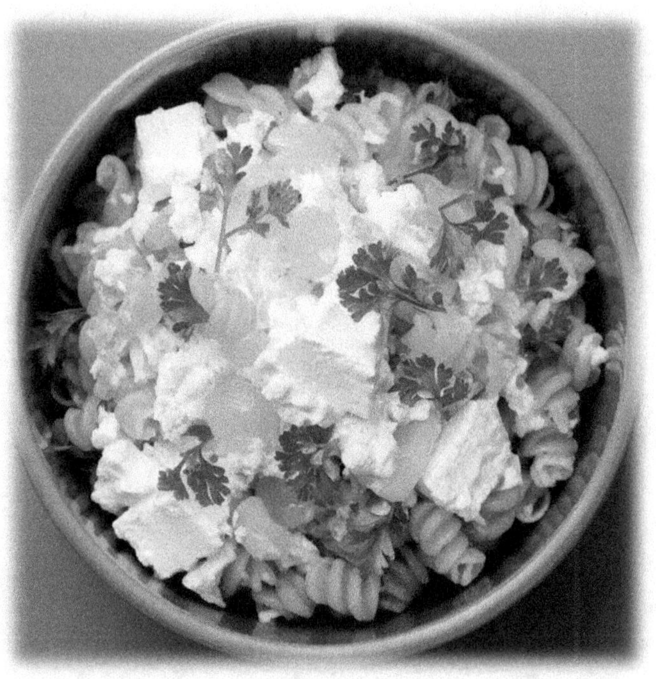

Ingredients:

½ cup of cooked scrambled egg

½ cup low fat cottage cheese

½ cup of cooked whole-wheat or brown rice pasta

1 tsp. finely chopped, fresh parsley

Instructions:

1. Scramble eggs.

2. Mix all ingredients together and serve chilled.

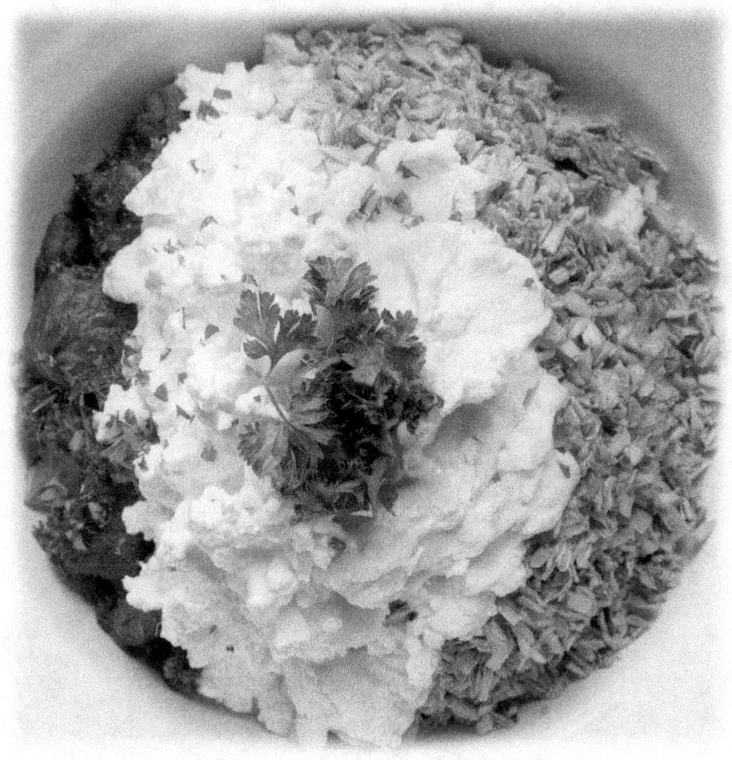

25. Poached Chicken and Brown Rice

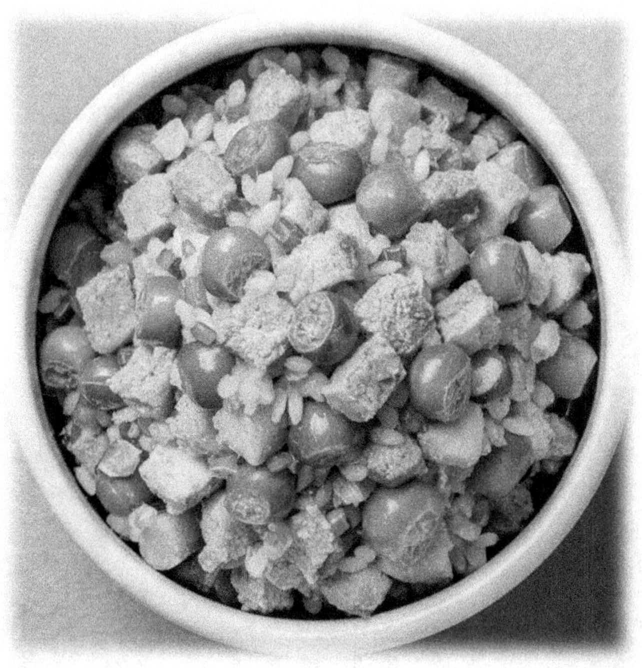

Ingredients:

1 boneless skinless poached, chicken breast

½ cup of cooked brown rice

½ cup finely chopped green beans

1 tablespoon of plain, low-fat yogurt

Instructions:

1. Soak chicken breasts in unsalted water.

2. Combine cooked brown rice, green beans, and yogurt to the shreds of chicken.

3. Serve at room temperature.

26. Baked Cod with Quinoa:

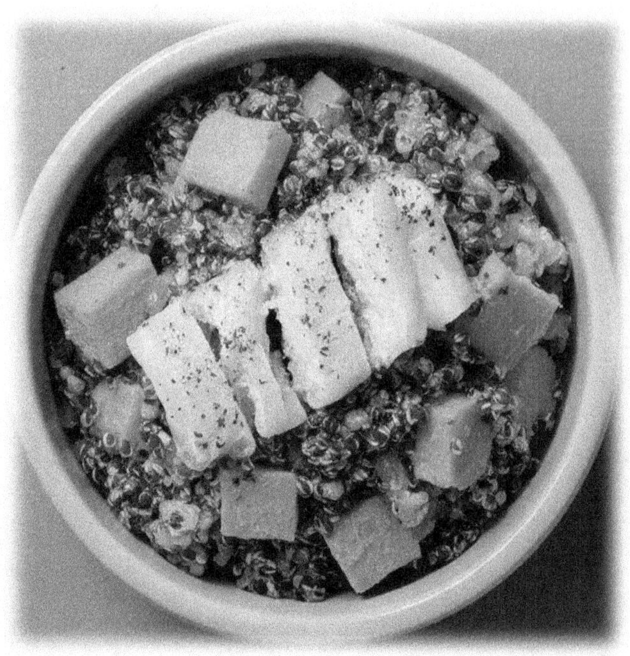

Ingredients:

1 baked cod fillet

½ cup cooked quinoa

¼ cup chopped roasted sweet potato

1 tsp. of coconut oil

Instructions:

1. Bake the cod fillet.

2. Flake cooked cod and combine with quinoa, roasted sweet potato, and coconut oil.

3. Serve at room temperature.

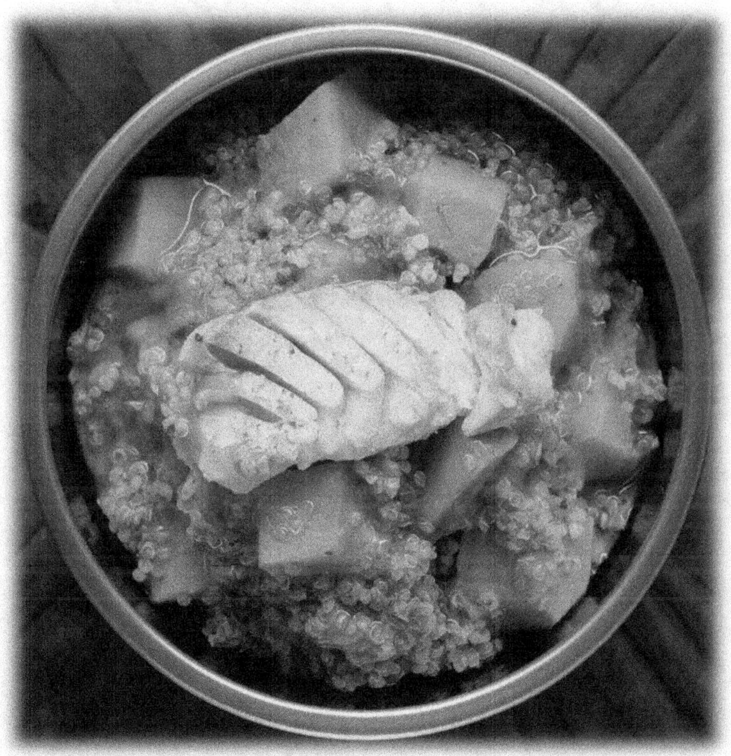

27. Scrambled Eggs with Vegetables:

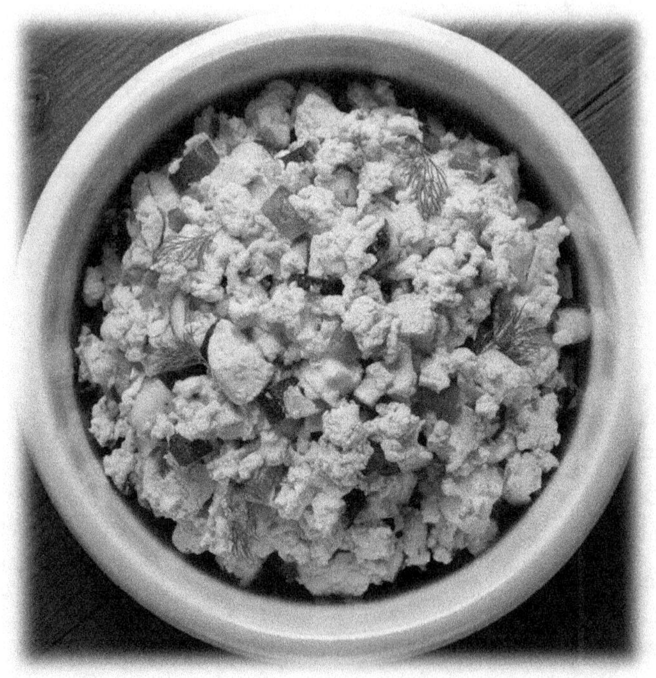

Ingredients:

2 scrambled eggs

½ cup of cooked chopped chicken breast

¼ cup finely chopped zucchini

1 tablespoon of freshly chopped dill

Instructions:

1. Scramble eggs.

2. Add chopped chicken breast, zucchini, and fresh dill to fried eggs.

3. Serve at room temperature.

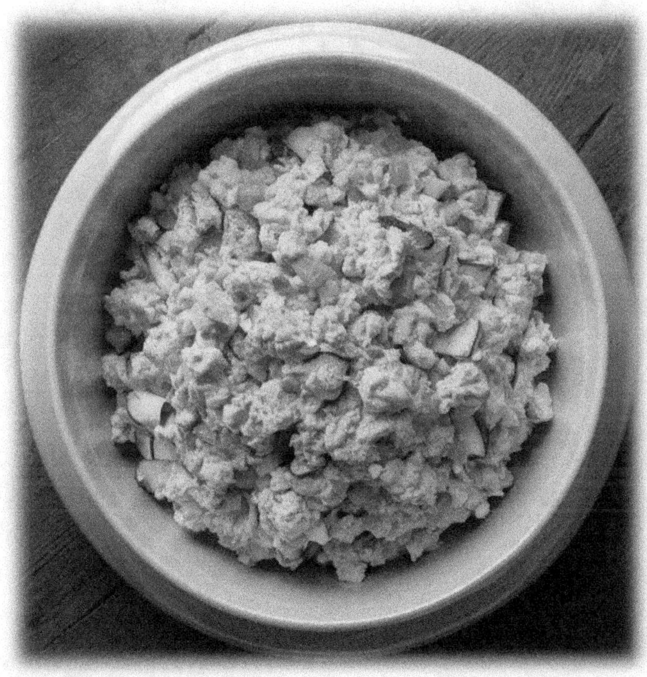

28. Turkey Meatloaf and Butternut Squash:

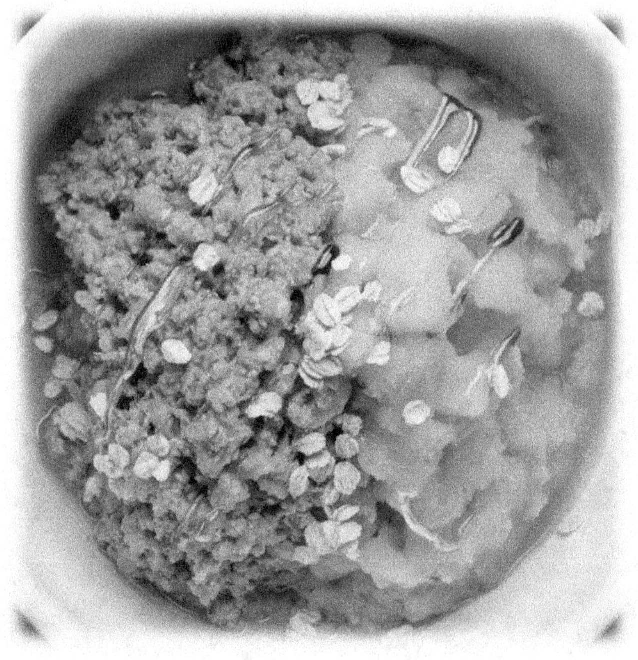

Ingredients:

1 pound of ground turkey

1 cup of cooked mashed butternut squash

½ cup of cooked oatmeal

1 tablespoon of olive oil

Instructions:

1. Set oven temperature to 175°C/350°F.

2. In a mixing bowl, mix together ground turkey, mashed butternut squash, oats, and olive oil.

3. Shape into a loaf and bake for half an hour.

4. Let it cool shortly before serving at room temperature.

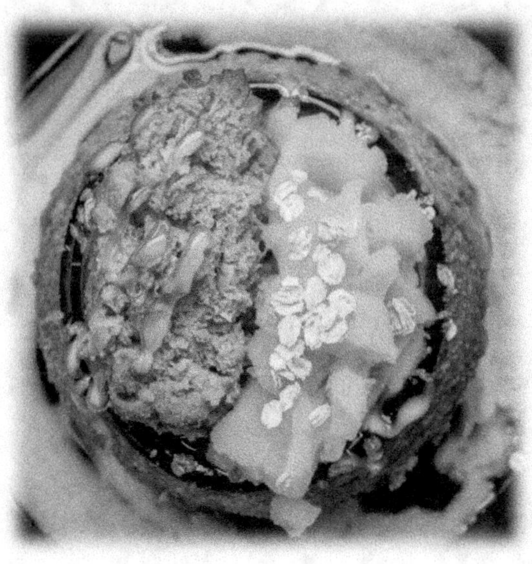

29. Turkey and Barley with Vegetables:

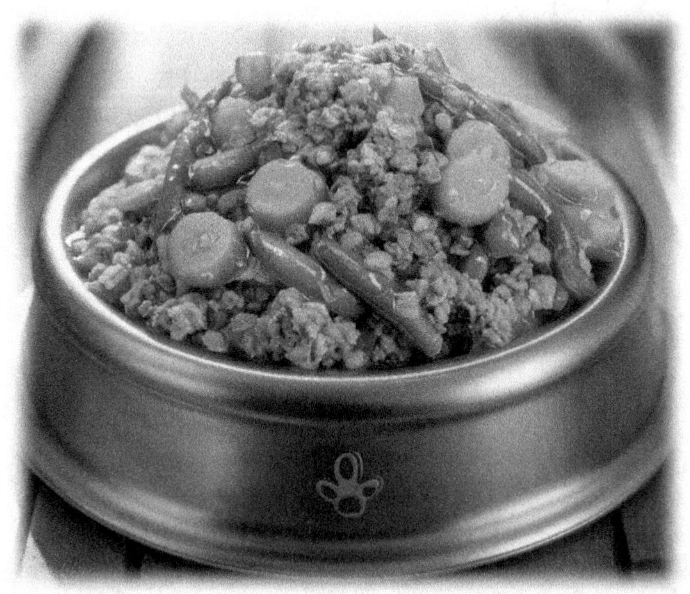

Ingredients:

1 pound of ground turkey

1½ cup of boiled barley

1 cup of finely chopped carrots

½ cup finely chopped green beans

2 tsps. olive oil

Instructions:

1. Set oven temperature to 175°C/350°F.

2. Cook the ground turkey thoroughly by sautéing it in olive oil.

3. Drain excess fat.

4. In a mixing bowl, mix together cooked turkey, barley, carrots, and green beans.

5. After spreading the mixture onto a baking sheet, bake it for 20 minutes.

6. Serve at room temperature.

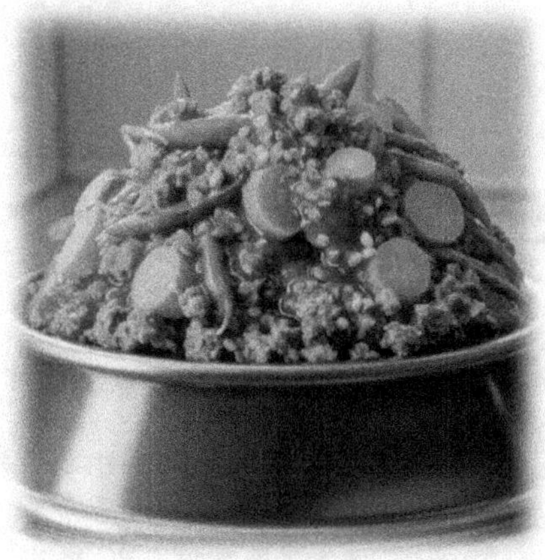

30. Salmon and Quinoa with Cottage Cheese:

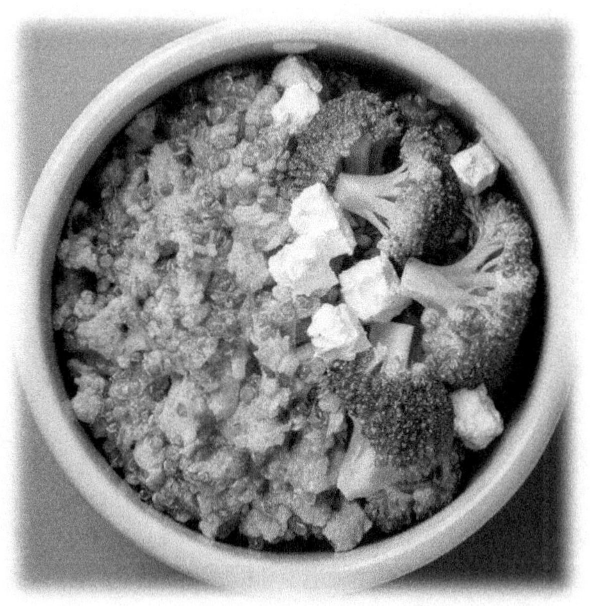

Ingredients:

1 cup of cooked flaked salmon

1 cup of cooked quinoa

½ cup of cooked chopped broccoli florets

¼ cup low fat cottage cheese

Instructions:

1. In a bowl, combine cooked salmon, quinoa, and broccoli florets.

2. Stir in cottage cheese and thoroughly mix.

3. Serve at room temperature.

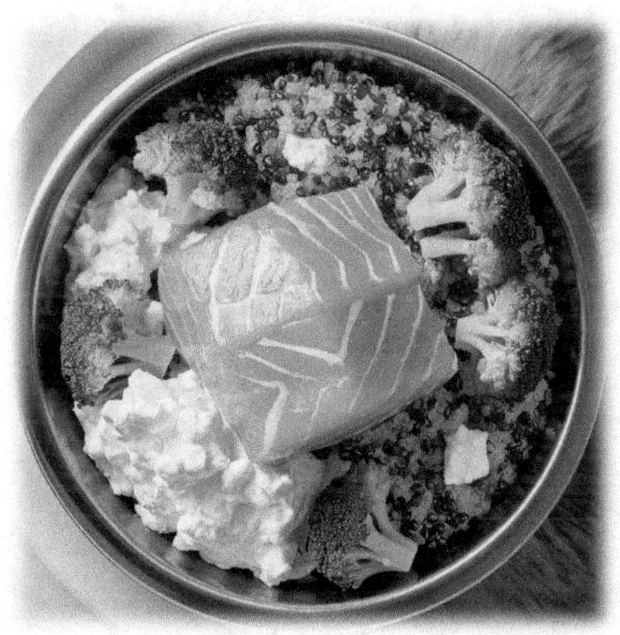

31. Chicken and Sweet Potato Casserole:

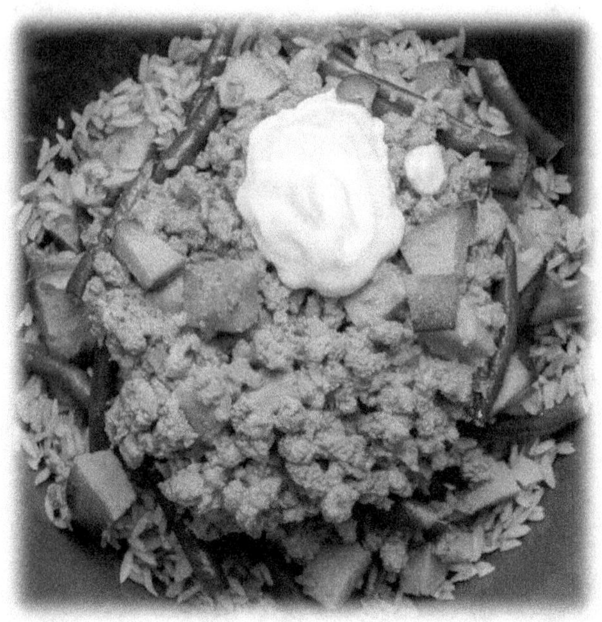

Ingredients:

1 cooked, shredded boneless, skinless chicken breast

1 cup of chopped cooked sweet potato

½ cup diced cooked green beans

¼ cup of cooked brown rice

1 beaten egg

1 tablespoon of low fat yogurt

Instructions:

1. Set oven temperature to 175°C/350°F.

2. In a mixing bowl, mix brown rice, green beans, sweet potato, and shredded chicken.

3. Add yogurt and beaten egg, and stir.

4. Spread mixture in a greased baking dish.

5. Bake for 20-25 minutes, or until thoroughly cooked.

6. Serve at room temperature.

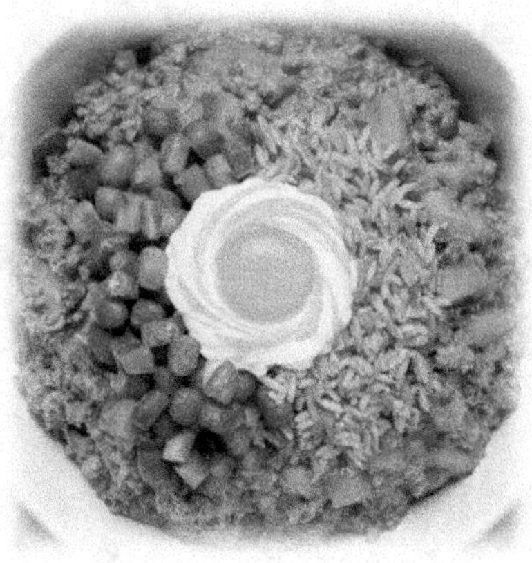

32. Tofu Scramble with Vegetables:

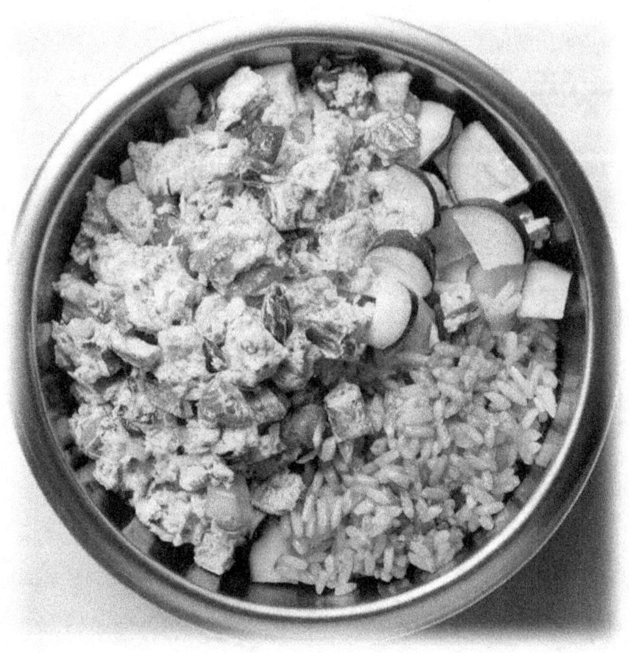

Ingredients:

½ cup cooked and seasoned crumbled tofu

2 scrambled eggs

¼ cup of chopped cooked zucchini

¼ cup of cooked brown rice

Instructions:

1. Scramble eggs in a skillet.

2. Add the brown rice, zucchini, and cooked tofu and stir.

3. Cook until well heated.

4. Serve at room temperature.

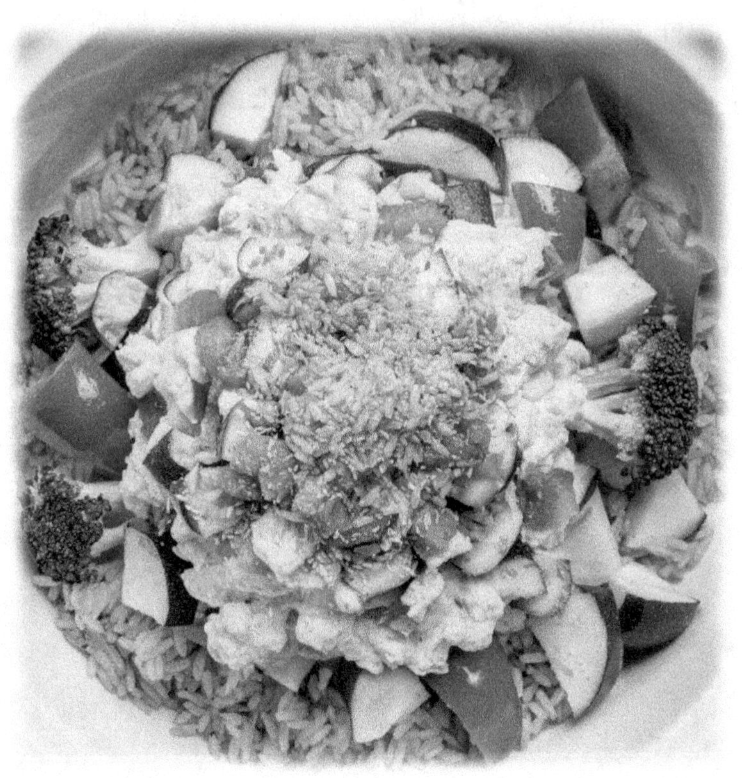

33. Baked White Fish with Lentil Soup:

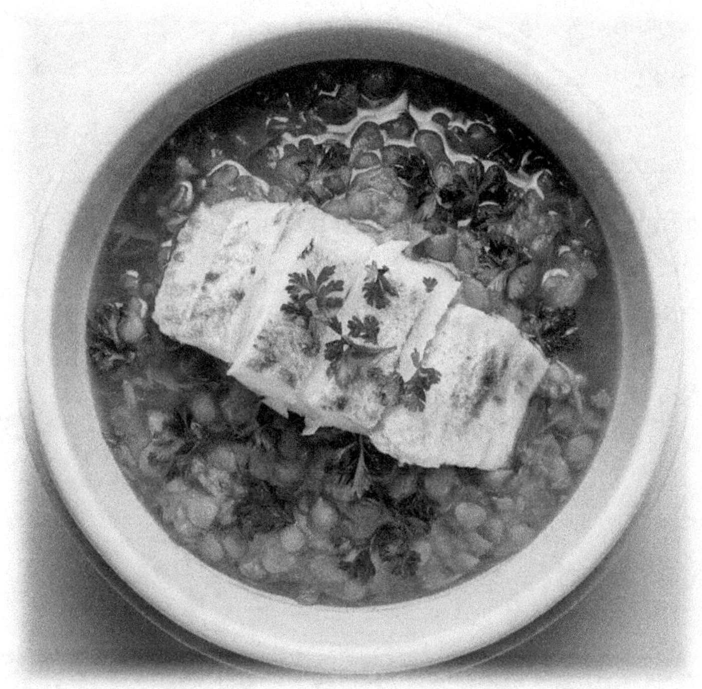

Ingredients:

1 baked cod fillet

1 cup of rinsed and cooked lentils

½ cup low-sodium vegetable broth

1 tablespoon of freshly chopped parsley

Instructions:

1. Bake the cod fillet.

2. Flake cooked cod and combine cooked lentils, vegetable broth, and chopped parsley.

3. Mash until a soupy consistency is achieved.

4. Serve at room temperature.

34. Scrambled Eggs with Chicken and Spinach:

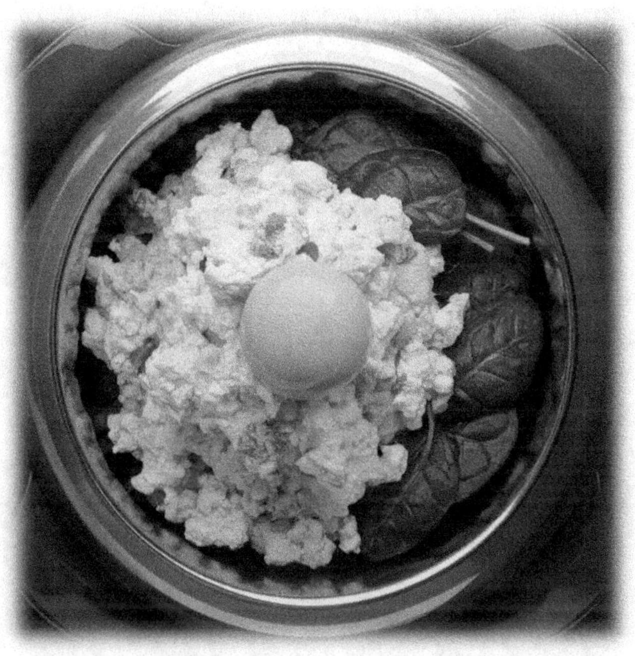

Ingredients:

½ cup of chopped cooked chicken breast

2 scrambled eggs

½ cup of finely chopped spinach

1 tsp. of coconut oil

Instructions:

1. Scramble eggs with coconut oil.

2. Add chopped spinach and chicken breast to cooked eggs and mix.

3. Serve at room temperature.

NB: Remove the egg yolk and cut the leaves.

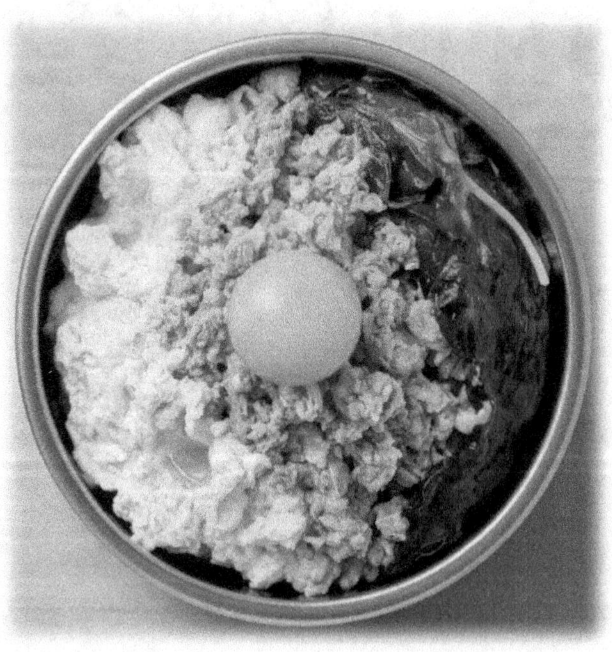

35. Salmon and Quinoa Salad:

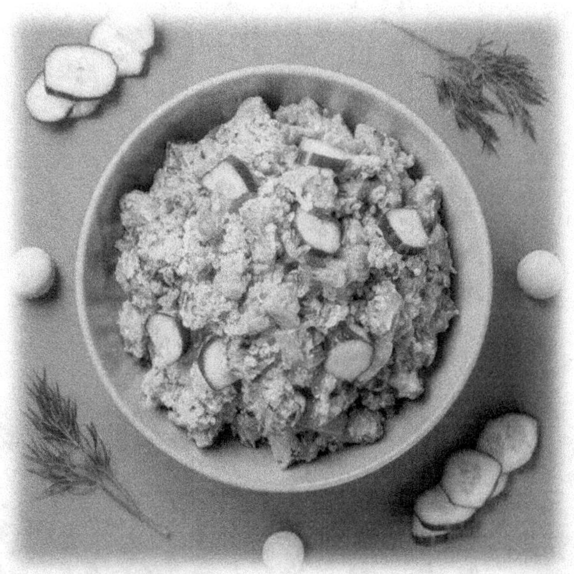

Ingredients:

1 cup cooked, flaked Salmon

1 cup of cooked quinoa

½ cup finely chopped cucumber

¼ cup of chopped fresh dill

Instructions:

1. In a bowl, mix cooked salmon, quinoa, diced cucumber, and fresh dill.

2. Serve at room temperature.

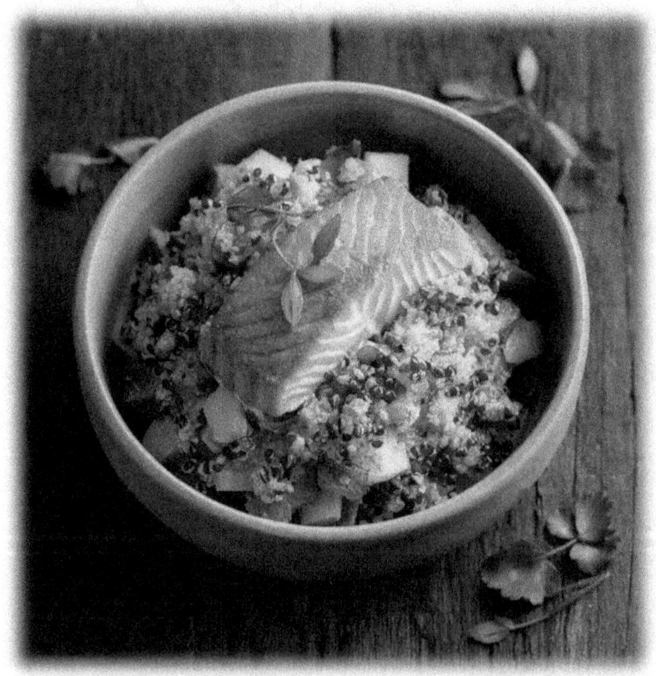

CONCLUSION

As we close the final pages of the "Pancreatitis Diet Cookbook for Dogs", it's my hope that you've found this book to be more than just a cookbook. It's a guide, a companion, and a resource in your journey to manage your dog's pancreatitis through diet.

We've explored the complexities of pancreatitis, its causes, symptoms, and treatments. We've delved into the crucial role that diet plays in managing this condition and the specific nutritional guidelines to follow.

But most importantly, we've shared a collection of carefully crafted, low-fat, and highly digestible recipes that your dog will not only love but will also help them thrive despite their condition.

Remember, every dog is unique, and what works for one may not work for another. It's always best to consult with your veterinarian before making any significant changes to your dog's diet. They can provide personalized advice based on your dog's specific needs and condition.

Thank you for taking this journey with me. It's been a privilege to share this information and these recipes with you.

Here's to many more happy, healthy years with your furry friend!

Keep cooking, keep caring, and keep loving.

Your Dog Is Lucky To Have You.